Alternating Your Mindset:

Perspective, Perception, Perceive

Michael C. Womack

Publisher's Name: Michael C. Womack

ISBN: 978-1-968442-12-5

Table of Contents

Chapter 1

The 3 P's Introduction

Since the beginning of man existing and interaction with the world civilization, development and interaction with each other there have always been the presents of three Ps. The thought processing of matters surrounding perceived, perception, and perspective is a profoundly serious social skill and self-management practice. The three Ps have contributed to many positive and negative events over the years. The results have contributed to many platforms, such as science, medical, legal concerns, and much more as people and the world continue to learn and develop. Those who as a group or induvial have learn to grow and make adjustment with their teams or individual goals to achieve great success, and in some cases, setbacks with adjustment to make a comeback or in other work forward progress due to gaining a better understanding of the situation or topic. Having the ability or even the skill set to master the recognition the use of the three Ps within any giving setting can provide you with a great gift to change or enhance situations or settings, including platforms enhancement that are under development.

The understanding of what we <u>perceive</u>, our <u>perceptions</u>, and <u>perspective</u> contributed to our world changes over the years in many, many aspects. During the early years, where man did not have transportation, comfortable housing, which includes climate control using current heating and cooling mechanical systems, is a lifestyle worthy of detail review to appreciate living conditions modernizations. This also includes how we should value and recognize in general how we decorate the interior finishes within our homes.

Decorations of your home is an outstanding offering of three Ps as you either assess your own home décor or that of others that you visit or have the pleasure to appreciate. A person home decoration offers opinions of their taste, such a hunter that like to post pictures of events or artwork mantels of animals as a show of artwork of their desire. In many instances, these types of decorations promote conversations that create positive social interactions.

Another example, which is quite common, are paintings in a person's home where the homeowner may share a variety of pictures that may consist of artwork posted in picture frames in a certain pattern or canvas paintings that may have a common blend with the surrounding canvas portraits. These paintings or pictures may be a capture of family, vacation trips, nature, or simply a means of showing one's appreciations for other art worthy expression. The wall decoration has created a landscape in the home and provide some sort of school of thought for a visitor to your home and an expression you are creating to share. This posting of artwork is a good alternative versus have nothing on the walls, which provide a blank three Ps observations. Some may walk away with a sense of troubling thoughts should they visit an established home that have no decorations. If you and that person have a relationship, you can anticipate some underline questions about how you are doing in general or try to pry to satisfy their understanding of questions as to why you have no form of expression or landscape on the walls. This can be off set with other forms of artwork, such as medium to upscale tabletop artwork which would provide a shift in their observations. Let us add to the home decoration landscape other visual aid that influences thought while the walls remain bare of artwork and add such different sizes of a statue with captivating designs. Designs that include eye catching materials while providing a charming presentation for your visitor. Imaging a blank wall that have an eight-foot tall five feet wide statue or even a nicely carving of the same size that is a design of your parents with a compromising wall paint color.

This concept of carvings or a statue interior décor landscape compared to a wall fill landscape of portraits pictures or canvas painting when compared to a blank and bare wall are providing three quite different conversation and affects a visitor's three Ps shape of notion to guide their feedback when they start to ponder and show interest with your decoration or lack of decorations.

Because of the thrive to flourish history have providing the world with a foundation of information and systems that have promoted growth and innovation. There were two major sparks that natured the global world history that made major improvements to way of life and mankind. Regardless of all the moving pieces that were involved with these two sparks the balance, negative and positive handing of perspective thoughts, perceived information, and perception outlook create a never changing insurgence on the way we live, work, and contribute to the economy. The two sparks were the Technological Revolutions (1950-1960) and the Industrial Revolution in the 19th Century.

During both revolutions, there were massive three Ps growth and systematic creations of methods to qualify quality measures while addressing the negative impacts of the two revolutions. In some degree to consider the Technological and Industrial Revolution created additional uprises, such as financial changes and improvements to banking systems were loans, interest rates, and record keeping processes become more of a focus with administration.

The technological revolution provided novel technology that create innovations cycles that accelerated progress. Basically technology was replaced with improved technology in a short period of time over and over. The required people to meet and complete review of three P chatter over and over to the point of agreement and implementation.

The industrial revolution provided a transformation from handicrafts and agriculture factoring into large scale mechanized industrial manufacturing production promoting efficient developments and programs. The transition from hand of man to machinery spread throughout the globe.

Both revolutions created a foundation of modern-day society. People became engaged with the new processes, programs, and general development. This promoted people to move from county side area to city and town development. The main drive was that as a society, work was being created so the workforce crew with the revolutions and now create another need urban study and development, including capitalism. The development of urbanization created government focus were as capitalism provided money making vehicles for creators and owners of business. Business owners needed balance vehicles, such as labor unions to address labor focus concerns and three Ps. The balance concerns are a tool to establish three Ps agreement and terms in order to move forward with agreed expectations between the labor forces and employers and continue to exist today, which is helping maintain positive attitudes, uphold promises, and address unforeseen concerns.

Aside from the revolution impact and growth of three Ps understanding another area, I like to touch bases on that is easy to relate with regards how we reside daily, in other words where we live our actual home outside of the decoration of our home is the construction efforts of homes over the years.

All these ideals of how we get from point A to point B have core raw sociology (functioning of human society) and philosophical (fundamental knowledge, existence of modern times) and these factors of elements have built us and caused us to buy into the civilization in addition to progress we enjoy today.

In the early 100 of years ago, the housing industry would consist of some form of construction that provide for the most part residential housing with construction materials that would not provide needed protection from the outdoor elements and the interior construction was constructed by craftsmen would provide skills sets that fasten material together to form chairs, tables, .and other needed residence use items. In addition there was no climate control that provide sufficient heating and cooling for the different seasons.

The standard homes would range in the area of 700 to 1,200 square feet with two or three bedrooms, no bathroom, and lack amenities that were not considered in the thought process during those early years, such as washing/drying machines, dishwasher, high speed internet, and other amenities in modern times that are in included in the amenity's categories note below:

Amenities by Category

Pet Amenities

- Pet-Friendly

- Dog Park

- Dog Washing Station

Transportation & Parking Amenities

- Garages

- Covered Parking

- Bike Storage Lockers

- Electric Care Charging Stations

Kitchen Amenities

- Dishwashers

- High End Kitchen Appliances

General Housing

- Air Conditioning

- Fireplace

- Patio or Balcony

- Storage Units

Technology Amenities

- USB Charging Outlets

- Smart Home Controls

- Wi-Fi

- High Speed Internet

- Cable and Satellite TV

Recreation Amenities

- Spa

- Yoga/Dance Studio

- Fitness Center

- Swimming Pool

- Playground

- Media Room

- Party Room

- Community Center & Classes

- Outdoor Areas (Jogging/Walking/Bike Paths)

Additional Amenities

- Security Cameras

- Security Guards

- Doorman

- Gated and Door Access

- Recycling Stations

As inventors gain momentum during the industrial revolution, they decided to dream and invent the expansion of what the perception for improving living conditions. That consisted of functional furniture, cooking conditions, sleeping arrangements, bathing comforts, then started to perceive ideas and test those actions and gain support for the perspective and conclude with results.-

Once the actual living conditions was shown to work and be functional, we humans have socially embrace the perspective of improve quality of living. The perspective for us now is unconscious that when you go into any home, the living conditions will provide you with quality in some form or degree with respect to interior standards, such as a bathroom, a kitchen, sleeping area, and other general living arrangements.

As humans we had the ideal of creating and combining the thought and action of the three Ps and create a more reliable and functional housing and residents, including climate control environment because of the three Ps. Most areas throughout the world have different cooling and heating requirements. Overtime these requirements have been studied (perceived data collection) to gain and achieved products and production means to support our experience with comfort because of the three Ps.

When the outdoor temperatures are below sixty-five degrees, you can go to your thermostat and turn on the heat and set a comfortable set point of seventy-four degrees, and within in a few minutes, your prospective is for your climate control desire and to achieve wishful or wanted design setpoint. The same is for cooling mode or set point. You expect to adjust your thermostat to let us say seventy degrees and expect to achieve temperature setting after a short period of time. When these temperatures do not meet your perception, and/or you not able gain your desire perceive comfort levels, you will want to investigate and understand what is at fault due to your perception is not met, your perspective and patients is being tested. This is a general ideal of why we want to understand the ongoing balance of the three Ps.

With respect to another paradigm or viewpoint, there have been major conflict over the years between individual or groups that resulted in positive or negative result because of either good balance of the three Ps or mis handling of the needed balance of the three Ps. Very often time it is needed to understand the message that is provided by the source (induvial or group). The information when taking out of content provide a negative perception, perceived wrongly, and promote a negative perspective. Now when the induvial or group are balanced in having a mutual understanding, the acceptance is received and promotes an agree to perspective, an agree to perception and united in what is to be perceived.

Now let us take in a couple case studies within one man's experience that is a generation of people experience that were bone in the 1900. This understand is a good example were the positive and negative three Ps shape history and provided an ever-lasting impact on society. These examples have details where the three Ps are present and were important factors that influence the desire outcome and influence the undesired outcome. It is especially important to allow your thoughts to break down the points of the three Ps and understand how perception, perspective, and what we perceive caused impactful changes and outcome on the subject matter. My/our example in the case study below will reflect an instance of a long-term and short-term historical situation and/or a systematic concept that is permanent fact in time.

For a small amount of perspective at this moment in history we are in; I imagine my great-grandfather born in 1900. When he was fourteen, World War I starts and ends on his eighteenth birthday with 22 million people killed. Later in the year, a Spanish Flu epidemic hits the planet and runs until he is twenty. Fifty million people die from it in those two years. Yes, 50 million.

When he was twenty-nine, the Great Depression begins. Unemployment hits 25 percent, global GDP drops 27 percent. That runs until you are thirty-three. The country nearly collapses, along with the world economy. Then Grandpa turns thirty-nine, World War II starts. He is still a noticeably young man.

When he is forty-one, the United States is fully pulled into WWII. Between his thirty-ninth and forty-fifth birthday, 75 million people perish in the war, and the Holocaust kills six million. At fifty-two the Korean War starts, and five million perish.

At sixty-four, the Vietnam War begins, and it does not end for many years. Four million people die in that conflict. Approaching his sixty-second birthday, you have the Cuban Missile Crisis, a tipping point in the Cold War. Life on our planet, as we know it, could well have ended. Great leaders prevented that from happening.

As he turns seventy-five, the Vietnam War finally ends. Think of everyone on the planet born in 1900. How did my grandfather survive all of that? A kid in 1985 did not think their eighty-five-year-old grandparent understood how hard school was. Yet those grandparents (and now great-grandparents) survived through everything listed above.

He was spit on in Georgia when he went to school. Now minority students are provided scholarships because of their ethnicity, athletic ability, and mental power.

Perspective is an amazing art. People must keep things in their appropriate perspective. We must be smarter, help each other out, be tougher, and we will get through all of this. In the history of the world, there has never been a storm that lasted. Our perspectives will lead us to victory or defeat. The entire group, including the grandfather experience form detail perception of today events, how all the historical events address economic matters were address with respect to the Great Depression, enhanced and modified to shape our business matters are handled during the 21ˢᵗ century. In addition how we presume matters is much different today than how matters were presumed in the 1900. Wars are fought differently as a result where technology have been designed to combat the situations and elements experience during the World War I and Vietnam War.

Lesson learned have shaped and develop best practices, design criteria, and other do and do not methods and approaches in order to achieve and maximize results as this related to business development, land use planning, technology, and even legislation. One of the most powerful attributes once fully understand by reading this book and developing your own three Ps understanding you ideally will start to find ways to advance your insight and enhance your decision-making concepts to improve in the areas of interest because you will have strengthened your ability to better influence how assumptions are shaped with respect to the subject matter.

The framework needed to assure that a project goals are met is a direct result of making sure you capture the desired perspective, address all good or bad perceptions, and achieve the desired potentials so that you minimize what is perceived by the general major of people or supporters. Common practices and standards are formed to address baseline gathering of information or establish baseline to start a project or subject matter is critical with control desire outcome of three Ps. To clearly help those readers understand examples of the importance of this book, introduction of the three Ps and all the important impact on our lives, I like to provide an additional overview of a legislative topic that is critical with designing criminal studies and programs.

There is an initiative underway where the FBI is reviewing its data collection platforms where all other state, county, towns, and local government input data regarding criminal cases could go away for one out of four police agencies. This subject is a large issue for Criminologist. Criminologists require data collection (perceived data) to determine measures and actions steps to combat crime that affect our society. These studies have strong insight prospective regarding perceived future conditions with respect to needed law enforcement management. Their work provides and identify common traits that assist us to better understand criminal behavior and prevent crime.

The platform is called the Uniform Crime Report (UCR) and now is being changed where platform at the FBI level will stop collection a limited amount of data from police agency. The police agency at the state, county, and local governments has their local challenges with being ready with the FBI platform switchover and change. As a result, the data collection will be reduced. The FBI UCR platform will not be able to capture crimes, such as domestic violence, rape, arson, and assault and battery from all police agencies. This will hinder reform practices and laws based on the report findings. This tool used by the criminologist impact how they can plan for better public safety. The comparison from community to community is extremely important for law enforcement.

Local police officers would not be able to get quality roll call briefing to improve the officer's attention and potential crimes during their shifts. The FBI will install a new platform call National Incident Based Reporting System (NIBRS). As we move alone with the three Ps concept and need to master the balance of the three Ps can you assure that new FBI effort, police agencies, and criminologists will enter a series of arguments and exchanges to improve the need of how crime perspective, perceived, and the public perception is impacted by the change platform of collection data for crime reporting into a central system. There may be a concern regarding the need for better transparency regarding the root cause of crimes that drive the need for data collection changes. The perceive overview understanding by the FBI is not in line with the general criminology community acceptance. It is safe to say that the three Ps will from a negative and positive dialog between the agencies to maximize the best outcome regarding public safety.

Very often the general concept or idea of a subject matter starts with one or more of the three Ps. As the element of support grows, so does the general outcome of the three Ps or even stop and regroup to next step the desired outcome of the subject matter (project, task, focus item etc.…). As part of human existing, the goal is to have long-term stability and growth. The effort to move forward require constant reevaluation of the three Ps and layers to review and develop the elements of one or more of the three Ps.

Throughout the world, because of the difference in views and to establish a universal acceptance of one or more of the three Ps policies, manuals, rules, and regulations have been created with detail focus to assure expectations and three Ps are understood and upheld to assure the desired general acceptance of a subject matter.

Throughout the book, the reader will start to shape a new understanding of the three Ps and how you will implement some sort of new way of conducting yourself within many different settings or platforms and excel with the overall self-development, goal-setting, or other desired outcome to gain success or advance the subject matter.

Because the world is very massive and large in far-reaching, you will find yourself in constant adjustment of your three Ps and the three Ps of others. This is where the start of discussion is formulated and become interactive.

Having the ability or even the skill set to master the recognition, the use of the three Ps in any giving setting can provide you with great gift to change or enhance situations, including platforms that are under development.

The situations may consist of conversations that be in a job interview or even a business or marketing meeting where you are working to make an impression to a client for a major deal or securing a raise. When you are in a leadership role or in coaching settings others, where you are require to provide guidance to achieve desire outcome your skill set and understanding with how to control the desire outcome and/or assumption of the desired outcome can be achieved with the knowledge to promote the accurate interpretation to gain expectations and provide the impression of success would provide you in every instance a pivotal experience and deciding moment to gain support of others including reaching your goals.

Mastering the three Ps is a skill set and a major fixed communication vehicle that will change how you conduct yourself in any setting moving forward. Your prior level of education will be improving, or your new learning will intensify your interaction on many levels with subject matters. It is ideally for the majority to find areas within ourselves to strengthen and make improvements. As you embrace the concept of this three Ps, you will agree that perception, perspective, and what we perceive is as old as time. This matter is a silent predominate function of communications, development, and root cause for change.

 Change is an ongoing need in society on many levels, in every family, in every government, in every business and economic growth throughout the world. Attention to detail alone with facts is a must to assure positive outcome, including having positive experiences with day-to-day activities versus negative results. As I work to bring focus to understanding and general awareness to this subject of self-development, I have found personally that if you promote avoidance or not accepting the full processing of how you are perceived, how perceptions are formed, and how perspective is giving birth and grow like wild grass, you will find yourself in some sort of recovery mode or lose your standing in that situation. This comment is more toward an individual or personal viewpoint. You can lose or have a setback in a group setting or teams format if you allow the three Ps to form a negative status that is controllable. You or the group will gain success if you can position the three Ps in a positive manner and sustain its establishment. This can be achieved by your self-development and mastering the art of controlling your performance and share this new skill set, which require your awareness and ability to make good judgment.

Educators have a standard way of providing information and learning skills to their students on all levels, ranging from K-12 through college and post college educational platforms. For the most part, the education you learn from a school or university setting will help you start your understanding at the foundation level all the way up to the professional performance level. At some point in your growth and career, the mastering of common sense and practical know-how of inserting positive management of perspective, perceptions, and perceive manipulation in a skillful manner will add massive value to your performance and confidence to handle matters. On the flip side, if you fall short with handling or controlling the flow of certain three Ps (perspective, perceive, perception) situation within your ability to administer, guide, or direct can cause you to recover work or form unwanted support of your time and effort, including have direct reflect on your image, which is important.

It is recommended that time is taking to understand the elements involved with the three Ps as these terms are old as anything else on this plant or universe. We are often familiar with the perception term in conversation or when issues arise. The one tip I like to offer as you accept, review, or choose to embrace the contents of this topic is that when you hear or speak of the perception term you include in your thought the other two terms (perceive and perception) to help with staring the process of skill set enhancement. By doing this overtime, your mindset will automatic start processing and references other instances to sharping your development. It may take some time for you to become aware of your self enhancement, which is natural. If you are mindful of the three Ps concept and complete back check reviews, which is a learning process, you will get there in a timely manner. Also, take note of others that may be already practicing this understanding.

It is a good practice to be open minded on all subjects to avoid having one sided perspective, so you can assure you are gaining well-rounded assumption of information that positions your perceived forthcoming belief. In addition it is to your best of interest to have a defined impression of what is shaping your perception as to what you are engage with or working through that is requiring your attention.

We are substantially knowingly or unknowingly introduced to need to process the three Ps on a high level in just about all that we do daily, in business, teams, and how we received information. The media world that consists of social media, television, literature, and general communication when we are talking provide us with an opportunity to practice how we shape and form our three Ps knowledge and development.

When you are interacting with others, regardless of the form, this is a perfect opportunity for you to start forming how you create your self-style with forming your practices of learning how to process information using the three Ps. It is acceptable and a good idea to take notes so you can follow up with how you wish to position your thoughts or research the topic. This will also enable you with how you position your plans to support or explain to others. Leaders are made by having a self-style to win over others and achieve success in the mass different areas of work areas or projects.

The success is measure by how you spend your time to achieve happiness, self-confidence, or monetary gains to name a few. If you are motivated and welcome this concept, you will discover new self-values by execution and comparing yourself with yourself. This means consider how you view yourself yesterday versus how you are developing yourself for the future. There are natural bias situations we are introduced to all the time. This is open and challenge us to be open minded while we process facts and cycle through your current three Ps mindset. The overall core goal is to achieve long-term results versus short-term satisfaction and not get either of the two twisted. So your three Ps development also help with avoiding getting subjects, conversations, or items you are working on with others distorted, tangled, or bent out of shape.

One of the great gifts to consider with appreciation time is taking the advantage to compare and learn from internal and external experiences. In modern times, access to external information by use of the internet is extremely useful. Testing your memory or ability to recall your past interaction with decision-making or observations will also aid your ability to master your own maturing and blossoming to make headway with good use and managing negative and positive influences indirect or directly with perception, perceive, and perspective.

Chapter 2

Identify the Difference

Prospective = Expected or Expecting

Percieve = Come to Realize or Understand (Data & Brain Stimulus)

Perception = Use of Senses to become aware of a state of something

Master the art of vetting information to gain the most maximum balance

Of what you expect, understand, and settle your senses in order to

Next, step the subject matter or express yourself through communications media.

In order to start the acceptance and master the mindset and thought breakdown of the three Ps, there is a full need to understand and define the difference of Prospective, Perceive, and Perception. Each of them has specific difference of understanding and blend with a topics, discussions, and variations within a subject or topic. Some of these subject matters related to positive or negative matters that could be related to an individual item, a team item, or a massive group involvement (teams) that may be working on a project, political matter, and needed agreement to next step an urgent subject matter, such as a time sensitive situation.

One of the cores and basics of accepting the three Ps understanding is that the existing of negative and positive must be capture during the thought process. The reason that the negative and positive comment is present is the fact that regardless of the subject matter, a plus or negative will be the outcome, and this will be the root to either next step the item of discussion or regroup on the subject of discussion, which could also be some sort of business matter. When you next step the subject matter, this is a result of positive outcome and understanding. When you have to regroup on a subject matter, this is a result or considered a negative subject matter.

On The Corner in Washington DC, A Man Appears to Be Homeless Due His Overall Appearance

After finishing up my morning with several meetings in a downtown DC office building, I decided to take a walk down the street to sit outside at a local sandwich shop. On this day, the weather was very comfortable with many people walking the sidewalk, going in and out of the many restaurants and sandwich shops. This was a great and ideal time for homeless people to solicit pedestrians for money during their lunch break. This is actually a very clever and straight forward time to capture the best ratio of people with money on hand due to either they are going to get their lunch and also is a good mental time to offer support to a homeless person. This concept within itself offer a general perception as the homeless community have their own perceive approach to receive donation from the general public.

I place my order for a turkey sandwich with a side of coleslaw and a medium iced tea to drink. While my order was being completed, I spotted a seat and the seating area where I would enjoy my lunch alone and people watch. I notice at the adjacent corner there was a man sitting on a white five-gallon container and with another five-gallon container open end up for people/pedestrians to drop their money for donations. The homeless man was a black African male, medium built wearing a solid black baseball cap backwards. He had on a black tee-shirt, blue jeans, and black sneakers. He had a beard and appeared to look tired. His overall appearance suggested to me that he was homeless due to the nature of the buckets and the flow of pedestrians making donations. There was also a medium-size black suitcase behind the homeless man that appeared damaged and dated.

As I continue to enjoy my lunch and people watch, the homeless man stood up and started to organize the buckets and the black suitcase. At this point, I was halfway through my lunch and really enjoyed my seating outside to refresh myself, returning to my office for the remainder of the day. The man in my review was not interested in making a clean physical appearance due to his rough beard, reversed hat, black tee shirt, and black shoes appearance. As he stood up, he then opened the black suitcase and reached for a stack of business cards. This caught my attention and started me to think what a homeless man is doing this for as he placed the business cards on top of the five-gallon bucket that he was seated on, which became a prop station for his cards for pedestrian to reach and grab the cards. As I continue to watch, I now see the man reach into the black suitcase and pull out what appeared to be a speaker with a cord. He placed the speaker next to the five-gallon bucket with the business cards. Now I see him pull an exceptionally clean brass coated and gleaming alto saxophone from this suitcase. This alto saxophone was extremely clean and shining. The sun light was very reflective from where I was seated and bounced off his instrument and promoted a very pleasant sort of light display that got your attention. He must have completed some sort of detail cleaning of his saxophone. I was like wow...Now I notice he pulls out of the suitcase a strap to attach to his saxophone. This strap was incredibly unique and had brass metals sewed onto the straps that created the appearance of class. The strap wrapped over booth shoulders and around his back. There are leather pads at the shoulder area that gave the strap an additional rich quality appearance. This was a tailored saxophone strap harness. Now I am starting to change my perception of this homeless man. The saxophone strap harness added a costume appears injunction with the gleaming instrument. The strap harness provided now what I am started to notice is a musician that is about to perform with his instrument. People continue to walk back and forth....I am fully focused on this man at this time as my perception and curiosity is peaking and want to hear him play this saxophone. As a young man growing up in Washington DC, I played brass and woodwind instruments in middle and high school. I must admit at this time my mindset has changed over the last ten minutes regarding this homeless man looking for donation to a musician solution for donations and advertisement. He now reaches inside the suitcase and pulls a small device and attached to the bell of the instrument. There were no wires....He now turns on the speaker...The speaker must be battery powered. At this point, I am really enjoying my observations. I decided to add desert to my lunch and got myself a medium vanilla shake to take back to my same seat. The man is now playing cadence on his saxophone as the sound is projecting from the speaker. The sound from the speaker was noticeably clear as the tone from the instrument was exceptionally smooth. The device attached to the bell of the instrument must be Bluetooth technology as there were no wires and the sound was clearly from the speaker. At this point, that black suitcase drew my attention even more as I said to myself this what appeared to be a worn, damaged, and dated suitcase was actually a well-designed mobile carrying case for his speaker, instrument, business cards, and other items he carries during his travels and perform out on the streets.

Now he starts playing his saxophone and have a very pleasant appearance with that gleaming instrument, custom harness that masked his black shirt. The blue jeans and black shoes are now not a focus as the music and relaxation of his dress make sense. The reverse hat and beard now make him appear acceptable and unbiased in thought. He was now a single band man playing his saxophone. As he continues to play his sounds out of the speakers were very soothing during the lunch period, and people are now starting to stop and listen. He sounded good and professional. He was professional when *you consider his total organization and light carry load of the two buckets and a well custom design black suitcase.*

Now I notice people are now taking his business cards from the card holder off the top of the bucket that he once sitting on...he had the entire bucket top filled with cards. My guess is that there were over a hundred cards. This also make sense, so he would not have to refill them as he continues to play.... He played a mixture of jazz, blues, soul, and current popular tunes. Now I am at the forty-five minutes point of my lunch break. I walked over, grabbed a business card, dropped a few dollars into the bucket, and return to my office. There were many people standing and listening to him play. I did hear someone say he was here for the last two weeks on Tuesdays. This was also a clever ideal as he can capture those people with his music, donation bucket, and business cards.

Once I return to my office and took a seat at my desk...I reviewed his business card. The card listed services for birthday celebration, dinner evening, wedding, and office events...The man was a true professional. The business card had a website, phone number, social media information, and list of events he will perform. I contacted him and had him perform at my 50th birthday party, and he was a pleasant hit for the event. He showed up on time with the same black suitcase and no buckets as had had a stage to perform and did not need his five-gallon buckets. I paid him $150 for two hours of service. The event started at 8 P.M., allowing people to show up for his start time of 9 to 11 P.M. His services were outstanding....He did a solo happy birthday musical that was a highlight of the evening. He passed out more business *cards and got more business. This was his living....Marketing himself on the street corners that he revisits and destined populated areas and had a simple customer approach and advertising...his gleaming saxophone and harness.*

My original perception was totally my own concluded thought and in error. If I would have picked up my lunch after seeing the homeless man sitting on the bucket with the black suitcase closed behind him and went to my office to enjoy my lunch while working or seated in the break room at work, I would have been left with that image of a homeless man soliciting for donation from pedestrians. Since I took a seat and continue to observe the homeless man and people watching my perception was reevaluated and became true that the man was a musician getting ready to perform versus a homeless man being idle.

Mining for Coal In West Virginia Provide Economic Growth for The State and Environmental Concerns.

Negative: *Erosion, Sinkholes Deforestation, Loss of Biodiversity, Use of Water Resources, Dammed Rivers and Ponded Waters, Wastewater disposal Issues, Acid Mine Drainage, Soil Contamination All Lead to Health Issues*

Positive: *Cheap Source of Energy, Provide Jobs and Livelihood, Land Made/No Import, Provide 56 Percent or More Electricity Source, Low Capital Investment, Huge Global Reserves, Simple to Store, Output is controllable, Risk are Easier to Mitigate*

The use of coal (combustible sedimentary rock formed by dead plants matter decay and converted to energy source after over millions of years) as a fuel source to generate energy started thousands of years ago taken on key importance during the Industrial Revolution of the 19th and 20th centuries, where it became a primary use for heating buildings, generate electricity, and source of fuel for steam engines. When compared to wood for fuel, coal provides a higher degree of energy per mass. In addition coal was universally used source of energy when compared with oil and natural gas due to its low need for engineering and design support with respect to production. Coal mining became a political and social issue since 1890 due to environmental issues, including health of miners, destruction of landscape, mountaintop removal, air pollution, and coal combustion when promote global warning concerns.

The Five Largest Coal – Producing States in The US Mining Technology Report 11/19/2018

- *Wyoming 297.2 Million Short Tonnes*

- *West Virginia 79.8 Million Short Tonnes*

- *Pennsylvania 45.7 Million Short Tonnes*

- *Illinois 43.4 Million Short Tonnes*

- *Kentucky 42.9 million short Tonnes*

The Five Largest Coal – Producing Countries Statistical Review of World Energy 2018

- *China*

- *India*

- *United States*

- *EU*

- *Australia*

As coal remains a resourceful fuel source and a key source of energy for production....etc.

Throughout the development of the coal mining industry,

the importance of the three Ps remain consent and remain adjustable throughout. I choose this subject of coal mining as an illustration of a broad and group overview of the three Ps, positive and negative outcome....

The coal mining industry has had many developments over the years that made improvements with tunneling, digging, and extracting of coal. These methods are net result of three Ps reviews that captured core understanding of Prospective (Planned of Improvement), Perceived (Data Collection), and Perception (Awareness & Judgement). Coal mining consist of surfacing mining and underground mining. Both mining methods require a set of rules and sub-line efforts by groups and individuals to assure production and safety in order to meet the world economic and environmental aspirations.

The Industrial Revolution was the period were the manufacturing process in Europe and United States in the period of 1760 through 1840 use coal as a fuel source for machinery production.

The world grew very dependent of this fuel source over the many years and created several support systems that involved groups, such as labor unions known as the United Workers of America (UMW or UMWA) in the USA the unit provide support for health care workers, truck drivers, manufacturing workers, and public employees. The UMN/UMWA was founded in 1890 with the merger of two old labor groups The Knights of Labor and the national Progressive Union. The labor union later revolved into a new group called the American Federation of Labor.

There are focus groups within the federal level that monitor concerns with coal usage, United States Environmental Protection Agency, and the World Coal Association.

Some consider coal mining is one of the most dangerous job in the world.

The two stories I shared provide a great degree of three Ps overview and content. The homeless man who was actually a musician provided a consent change and balance of the three Ps. I could have simply concluded that this man was a typical homeless individual on the streets of Washington DC with no goals or meaningful lifestyle. What took place was unique and need to be captured and understand the importance of vetting information. I was able to vet my own observation due to my mindset and the environment of my surroundings. The weather was inviting while having lunch and people watching. People watching by itself of others is a form of your unknowing processing of the three Ps. Very often when you people watch, you toy with the throughs of prospective, perception, and what you perceive. We watch people and gather data, such as dress fashion and styles including how people interact with each other, whether you notice specific demeanors or negative demeanors. The observation of the homeless man, which who was a particularly good musician, is a positive three Ps item.

The overview provided regarding the coal mining industry is a positive and negative subject that is ongoing and is revolving all the time due to a much broader three Ps content. Over the many years, organized groups, individuals have shaped the industry because of what is known information regarding prospective. The data collection has enhanced perceived information and the sense the coal product itself, have established a well understanding of perception of use and use of the resource. The industry is a global share responsibility to keep workers safe, improve environmental impact, and economic upkeep. Because of the need for the coal resource over the years, the need to address conflict promote negative and positive three Ps were as the positive out weight the negative impact in the short-term. Due to the need to find other means of energy and remove fossil fuels from the equation, the opposite applies to the long-term with negatives out weigh the positive concerning the use of coal and mining efforts. Currently world is focus on renewable energy options with the intent to remove coal use at some point in the future. The intent by all involved is to minimize the negative impact while the world benefit from the positive impact of coal production and usage.

The exercise and tasks related to choosing the positive of the three Ps and managing the negative of the three Ps is my understanding in this book that need to balance three Ps. This terminology requires a skill set and deep understanding for the reader and is my desire outcome to help enhance yourself develop with processing information and formation your acknowledgement.

Self Three Ps Skill Set – Understand the Negative & Positive Three Ps Balance (Management) Equation.

Perception Overview

Prospective Overview

Perceived Overview

Now let's review the difference of the three Ps while keeping in mind and the thought process that is foremost principal of how to master and balance the concept of these aging and ongoing subject. In addition the balance remains the knowledge and viewpoint of sociology and philosophical outlook. The influence of one's interactions with others in any of the settings (business, technology, etc....) remains diverse and cause for understanding and separations within the content of Sociology and Psychology.

In order to shape this understanding before defining the three Ps, let's review a political topic that require balance of the three Ps while understanding the interaction of Sociology and Psychology.

Currently throughout the world, we are in a very historical and challenging period dealing with the reality of the Covid-19 pandemic and aftermath. The pandemic has caused an array of issues that relate to economic step back/downturns, health concerns which relate to chronic stress, anxiety, depression, alcohol/drug dependence, and massive lockdown scenario resulting to unemployment in all affected countries. In addition was the mass health officials and leaders of the different organizations throughout the world address the many elements of the pandemic, they also have to be flexible and address the fact that this issues is constantly changing matters that is profoundly affecting lives around the globe.

The handling of the pandemic, how to resolve, and manage the outbreak of cases, address the death rates, and support the health officials and front line health care providers have grown to be a major political matter that tests the need for powerful leadership. In the different countries, there are difference with how current leaders and change of hand with leadership are selling themselves, planning, and forward vision projection to address and provide a positive outcome to establish the new norm for the pandemic and assurance for the future outbreaks deterrent and measurement. Currently the current new norm present huge concerns and open-ended issues.

The three Ps is front line and center with how current leadership and the change of to the new leadership will handle the multiple issues and needed support for or to gain a positive outcome of the globe pandemic issues and learn from the negative impact of the pandemic. Their views and how they can influence what have been learned from the data collection is a direct future projection of what to perceive and determine what is forthcoming. There have been substantial learning and shaping of the desired outcoming in some cases because what was perceived and now uncovered. There has been meaningful enhancement with their judgement due to leadership experiences have shaped their perception with how they may gain support of their views and promote arguments for support. As these leadership move forward to be elected for their desired positions, the prospective will need to gain support by means of rallies, commercial advertisement ads, and internet platforms to provide insight details of their plans.

Perception

Common Quotes

"Perception is reality or is reality perception?" (A)

Perception is an individual or group viewpoint of as to how they view reality. Perception is extraordinarily strong with how impressions cause you to focus and remember a subject matter, including how you understand and decide on the reality of the subject matter...

Perception also unknowingly caused many times assumptions and overestimates of information or output of your thoughts.

One should also ask themselves, "Can I trust my perception?" (B)

Let's be straightforward...Very often perception is a design effort to gain attention with underline goals. (C)

Attachment of Style, (D)

Define and discuss Transference of Feelings. (E)

Mind Mapping (F)

Mirror, Mirror (G)

(A)

*Very often people or situations dictate a thought or concept of understanding that either holds true or require reevaluation. These thoughts or concept of understanding can be a physical observation, a want to hear or accept the subject matter, or a simple lack of vetting of information. In many instances the impression you received on a subject matter promote and starts the foundation of how you start to root your perception and formulate the mental position that you will start to support and promote your judgement. This entire way of thinking is an unconscious formation of thought that lead to how you will vocalize or take action on your perception.

For instance let's look at an observation example where perception was concluded and reevaluated and notice how this process holds true with the fact that perception is a natural ongoing subject that take on particular bases that are either true and false conclusions. This conclusion is the needed result to establish the correct next step and needed closure of the subject matter in order to solidify and settle on the end result.

(B) One should also ask themselves, "Can I trust my perception?"

We as individuals are entitled and have the right to have our own thoughts and conclude on what we believe vetted or not in order to be move alone with our perception on a subject matter. This is also the same thought when working within a group that is focus on a common goal.

(C) Let's be straightforward…Very often perception is a design effort to gain attention with underline goals.

Marketing is a great example of a design effort to gain attention to increase sales or gain interest for potential business. There are also incentive insert to encourage your perception of on a subject matter. The of promotional literature, mass media advertisement are forms of design perception.

(D) Attachment of Style

Branding came of age. Air Jordan, McDonalds

(E) Define and discuss Transference of Feelings.

(F) Mind Mapping

(G) Mirror, Mirror

Prospective

Common Quotes

" Prospective Is Also Known As One's Truth" (A)

Prospective is a combination of the present condition or thought while having the outlook and view point the forthcoming and or future condition or possibilities. When defining the term, one must also consider concept forthcoming, such as projections, potentials, and anticipated results.

Discuss game planning in sports, pre-screening platforms marketing etc..use of prospective. (B)

Prospective vs Perceive Define the difference (C)

Degree of Difference -DOD (D)

Impair our ability to solve problems (E)

Open to Rework Information (F)

Sensation Transference (G)

" Prospective Is Also Known As One's Truth"

Discuss game planning in sports, pre-screening platforms marketing etc…use of prospective.

Prospective vs Perceive Define the difference

Degree of Difference -DOD

Impair our ability to solve problems

Open to Rework Information

Sensation Transference

Perceive

Perceived is the verbal (verb of action) action of becoming aware or to recognize the particulars of a thing or subject matter. Very often what is perceived is based on a form data collection

Data Collection

We like market research because it provides certainty – a score, a prediction: if someone ask us why we made the decision we did, we can point to a number.

When you are in the product development world, you become immersed in your own stuff, and it's hard to keep in mind the fact that the customers you go out and see spend very little time with your product.

Groups

- Industrial Designers Society of America

- General Support of Concept

- Pricing and Marketing

- Chair Design

- Branding Things

Chapter 3

The Presence of 1,2,3

The presence of the three Ps can be physical, invisible

(assumption), psychological/influenced, smell, touch,

Taste, sight, sound,

I enjoy going into my garage to prepare myself for a nice open-air bike ride in my neighborhood or load my bike onto my vehicle bike rack to travel to a bike trail. There is a very enjoyable bike path in the Severna, Maryland area that provides a nice scenic course that travels behind residential homes, wooded areas, and there is a row of stores that accommodate bikers so that you can stop, park, and enjoy ice cream, a drink, and sandwich shops. This trail is also a perfect trail to ride when you as a cyclist like to keep the ride level without a challenging terrain. The course has several miles of flat non-hilly trials that promote a smooth ride that even encourages coasting, which is also a pleasure for some bicycle riders. If you are a cyclist, there are times where you like for your bicycle to take smooth lengthy coasting without the need to focus pedaling, climbing, or controlling your speed as you descend a hill to maintain a clam distance from other bikers, walkers, and children that maybe out enjoying the trail.

On this day in the summer, as I road my bike going south on the course, my three Ps were at a heightened calm. My energy was remarkably high and positive. I felt if I could ride for hours. The temperature was roughly eighty degrees with no real humidity which provided me with no sweating and low self-energy use while paddling and coasting during my ride.

My pre-prospective of the ride provided me with a great deal of joyful thoughts as I wanted to get a smooth ride in for the day so I can reflect on my achievement of adventure, fitness, and simply enjoy the outdoors on this great summer day.

My perception was in line with my effort for the day as I wanted to have a ride that I can anticipate my environment and repeat the surrounding enjoyment that I am familiar with for this trail. I have travelled this course before, so I had a comfort level as to what was before me from the un-racking of my bicycle returning to the rack for the ride home.

My perceived ride was also foreseen because I had no doubts of the terrain that further enriched my ride because anticipation.

The entire ride has always been a pleasant and delightful three P experience.

As I continue my ride, the engagement of three out of the five human senses are actively proving the ride with direct relationship of my surroundings. These three human sensing organs provide your brain with the presence of three Ps automatically and give you a sense of trust and confidents, which contribute to your enjoyment.

The use of your smell, sight, and hearing is a way of receiving the presence of the three Ps daily and during your travels. At this point, let us not include taste and touch as I am trying to provide focus on your casual recognition of being aware at all time of your ability to notice the presence of one, two, three (three Ps). The order in which you process prospective, perceived, and perception is interchangeable and use of your three senses of smell, sight, and hearing. Your mind will naturally cycle through the sequence of the three Ps if you acknowledge the human senses that are present to your while you process thought. One of the great gifts of the human senses that you do not normally think about is how the brain processes your human senses.

Sight is perceiving things through the eyes.

Smell according to researchers over time a human may be able to smell over 1 trillion scents.

Hearing provides audio perceptions and the ability to perceive sounds.

There are times where you may focus on sight to gather your three Ps, and the same will apply to your smell or hearing. Based on your maturity, you can determine which one of the three Ps you will place in order to evaluate, study, or inspect information. A young person will process his three Ps much different than a teenager, and an adult will process their three Ps much different than the youth in theory. I say in theory because we must leave room for those that choose or fail to catch on to the fact or reality of information or conditions that they may be involved with or situations. For the most the major would agree that education is an important part of our society, which is supported on a large scale by the government on all levels in the many cities, towns, states, and country thought the world. One of the intents of education is to provide discipline of your three Ps and boost your skill set in common needed areas of study.

Education brings an instinctive and long-lasting change in a person's ability to reason and achieve objectives. Education helps us to investigate our own considerations and thought processing and shape our various topics. It also helps us to distinguish the negative and positive causes of topics. This development contributes to self-enhancement with respect to your frame of mind. Believe it or not, we owe it to our self to grow with having proficiency and awareness with processing our surroundings by teaching our self the presences of one, two, three and the sequencing of the information provided by our smell, sight, and hearing. Once you built this into your personality, you will have create great powers. Thought education vehicles and platforms alone with your experiences, this development can be completed.

There are three types of education – Formal, Informal, and Non-Formal

Non-Formal Education

- Learning from Experience

- Learning at Work

- Learning from Home

- Learning through process or process learning

- Learning from your environment

Formal Education

- Certification or Degree

- Schools or Institutions (K-12 and Higher Education)

Informal Education

- Real Time Exposure Learning

- Local Resources

- Adult Learning Programs

Again the order (presence of one, two, three) can alternate based on how you prioritize perception of the topic, perceived of information provided to you, and how your prospective of thoughts shared or your own core feelings. We all know it is to the best of our interest to be aware of the environment and circumstances, including the condition and objects that are in our immediate zone. We typically like to process in our minds what is going on around us within eyesight. When looking forward, we like to focus forward vision and take time to look side to side at times. For some of us, we practice rear vision also to get our prospective, perception, and perceived details, then quickly process our thoughts and reset our mindset in order to be satisfied with our zone (surrounding area) and comfort level.

Our comfort level simply means avoidance of being uncomfortable and self-assurance of being at ease and content with your well-being. This also means having a physical complacency of your environment.

Below is a sample sequence order of how you may process your three of five human senses while you go about your day-to-day life and obtain your presence of awareness of your environment within your control.

Sample Order:

  - Smell, Hearing then Sight

  - Smell, Sight then Hearing

  - Sight, Smell then Hearing

  - Sight, Hearing then Smell

  - Hearing, Sight then Smell

  - Hearing, Smell then Sight

These are straight forward six combination of how quickly you can be aware of your process of the three Ps while moving about your day-to-day activities. This can also apply when you are in a group setting. In order to get the most information and your presence of the one, two, three format, it is best to be a good observer. By doing this first, this allows your mind to capture intake information and settle your thoughts by adding up and establishing facts about the presence of what is being observed. At this point, you will have form your mindset and qualify what you have chosen to accept and categorized. The human senses are under used if you practice avoidance behaviors of your natural three senses we are reviewing at this time.

As I continue to ride my bike, I for the most part focused on front and side to side vision to understand part my overall experience and appreciation of the sights, hearing, and smell (Presence of one, two, three in combination). As I approach a cross intersection where it is important to slow down and acknowledge a bike trail stop sign due to car traffic that cross the trail at this point and the vehicle traffic has the right of way. I must accept this in my processing and be responsible and socially correct, so that there will be avoidance of injury to myself and of others as we do not want a setback to myself and people that I am crossing path with on this great day. Therefore my sight is important as I approach this intersection alone with the other people who are enjoying their day out on the trail. We all are sharing a common interest to be observant and make use of our sight.

Now that I have completed my stop at the stop sign, I now proceeded further along the trail and continue to enjoy my ride safely. I kept up with watching other cyclists, runners, and children that were on the trail alone with stops at other intersections where stop signs were posted. For the most part, as a trail user, the stop signs were far apart and make for great continuous riding.

After riding for about forty minutes, I am now approaching the row of food and beverage outlets that are very conveniently positioned alone the trail. As I approach, my sense of smell was now playing on my mindset to take a break and enjoy a snack and drink. The odors from the exhaust fans provided the air with inviting smell of gourmet type of foods availability to try and advance my thinking to stop all because of the smell of food. This is a refreshing confirmation of being influenced by the presence of the three Ps alone with my sense of smell. My mind told me to take in the smell, stop and enjoy something while I take a short break. My discipline also had to kick into my mindset during my stop. I could smell a bakery, burgers, and steaks, which all were too heavy of a food intake for me to consider at the moment.

Inserts Rails to trails course markers, stations looks in the early 20th century, end in Annapolis at the Navy Academy.

Multi Use Trail and Fitness Trail

My goal for the ride was to enjoy myself and gain some level of fitness exercise for the day. I could not let my lack of discipline due to smell override my goal. So I made a health choice and ordered a low carb fruity smoothie and a fruit cup. I took a seat at an outside table and enjoyed the environment. My bike was safely parked on a rack and all secured. My break lasted twenty minutes; during the entire time, the smell from the exhaust fans were challenging. I promised myself I would enjoy a good dinner later to offset my mindset that was being guided by my sense of smell. *Laugh Out Loud -LOL Self Promises are AlWays Good...* My since of sight remain calm and enjoyable as I was seated at the table and observed people and cyclist moving about the area. Also, on the street side in front of the row of outlets were normal street traffic, which offer another set of environmental observations.

As I started to ride my bike, I now like to focus on the third element of the presence of one, two, three, which is hearing. I could hear voices of parents taking to their children on the trail...Such as "Honey, Watch Out...Move to Your Left" or "Honey, Stay in Your Lane" to help the kids stay aware and practice their own needed development of prospective, perception, and perceived understanding while on the trail that is being share with others. This is a particularly important area of focus for children and a huge part of their development. Can you image a child growing up and not gathering their development of the three Ps later on into their teens or adult life? The fact that I notice parents on the trail with their kids talking and I can hear them giving direction and the kids responded to their parent's direction is a priceless development. The opposite would be a young kid with a bicycle riding in a large yard in the county or rural area while riding, they do not get to interact with sharing of the road or bike trail. No fault to them because of where they are and enjoying that ride away from others...they miss out with sharing and processing broader surroundings and development.

Another sight item I like to offer during my bike right was the scenery. This ride offers a good sense of community, family, social connection with strangers, safety, and history. The trial course **(Baltimore Annapolis Trail/Rails to Trails Thirteen miles)** offers historical information for an old abandon railroad track system. There are statues and reading information alone the trail that gives you a prospective about the rail to trail history and past. Much like when you visit some towns, which have or provide museum type of data and you find yourself reading the pedestal signs.

All of this atmosphere is a much-needed positive presence of the three Ps. There were no negative three Ps to share, and when I repeat my ride on this course, it is the same every time. The route of me sharing the bike ride experience on this trail is an example where we all like to have a comfort level as to what we want to anticipate or have a comfort level on our outlook as we go about have an adventure, bike, or even a jog or run. I am safe to say that a runner or jogger share the same three P comforts when they choose a course to run or jog. The idea is to have an advance apprehension what is present, so that you can have a sub conscious settlement as you go about your journey. If there are negative concerns with your sub conscious understanding, then your thought regarding an acceptable presence of one, two, three would not be enjoyable to you and you will adjust. The opposite would be a negative presence of one, two, three where you have an uncomfortable level regarding your jog or ride because the presence of your sight, smell, or hearing is overly concerning and uncomfortable during your ride, jog, or walk. Since we are using the bike trail in this perception, let's change the setting to alter a positive presence of one, two, three to a negative presence of one, two, three, and as a reminder, the three P's can come in any order based on what is present or in front of you in real time.

Also, you must consider a negative ride is an opinionated thought based my comparison of the trail I experienced and enjoyed. I say opinionated because of preference, as I like a calm, steady ride without a lot of traffic and distractions. I am ok with the occasional family interactions, walkers, and the feel of shops and stops along the ride. If the trail was let's say much different, such as in the heart of New York City, alongside the Hudson River or the Lake Champlain bike trail where the course is surrounded by water on two sides. The Lake Champlain trail is very isolated with a rough pebble rock surface and remote whereas the New York City trail is busy with people and the surface changes often from pavers to concrete to asphalt to wood planks. For me and my presence of the one, two, three, either would be extremely uncomfortable because I have experienced and know that the Severna Maryland Trail do not present these discomfort and challenges. Now if you are a New Yorker and you are used to this condition, you are much more tolerable of the trail terrain changes and all the items that play on your personal smell, sight, and hearing. You would need to bare the sounds of heavy traffic, construction work, and the smell of the city and sights of all the tall buildings and Hudson River. Also, in New York, biking/cyclist present bike lane concerns, city laws are different than other cities, more hazards, and you need to be mindful of other dangers, such as if you have a nice bike will you be approached. The Lake Champlain ride requires you to be very well-prepared for bike repairs, restroom stops, and wind impact due to the isolation of the trail. As you can see, the three different trails offer many different demands of an individual readiness and willingness to accept the presence of one, two, three of that particular bike trail.

The core point here is that everyone has a different sense of knowing what you are around and how your senses (sight, hearing, and smell) react or do not react. You also need to consider simple matters, such as when you need to walk my bike. Yes…this is a fact when you enjoy riding your bike or cycling. There are times when you will need to walk your bike, and this happens a lot in New York during periods of high density with people or other objects. My experience in my local area and the trials I choose, I never have to walk my bike due to the elements that the other two trails present. Nor will I have to labor some of the issues, such as pebble dust from the Lake Champlain trail. You will also use your bell or whistle a lot in New York and almost none on the Lake Champlain trail. Also in New York when mentioning more traffic, you will find scooter, skaters, and skateboard users. Please note that I am only mentioning the bike trails, not the bike lines on the roads shared with cars. The shared roads and bike lanes on the roads present a totally different set of challenges and presence of one, two, three and avoidance regarding your ability to stay active with your three Ps.

Let's review some interesting features of the three different bike, jogging, fitness trails just to point out how important it is to appreciate individual preferences and make use of available resources. This thought is also an effort to recognize how the degree of differences with your senses and enjoyment are flexible with respect and an individual's comfort levels. Your comfort levels are also influenced by how your character is positioned at the time of your desire to go out onto one of the three trails.

The first trail, Baltimore Annapolis Rail to Trail, provided a scenic route that was a railroad course that traveled behind homes in a wooded area surrounded by flowers, residences, shops, and man-made stop designed for fitness use. The rider can simply enjoy a calm cruise.

The second trail, New York Hudson River Greenway, provided a busy and congested course along the Hudson River that is highly populated with people, buildings, and major city activities. The rider must stay alert and process data at a high rate.

The third trail, Lake Champlain Trial in Vermont, that provides a very isolated pebble course surrounded by water on two sides. The course is somewhat narrow and allows for no mistakes with crashing due to large rocks used to outline the course. Also, the course has this open feeling that keeps your attention honest regarding that you want to avoid going into the lake at all costs.

Again this comment amounts to self-preference and access. For me personally…since I have access to the railroad to trail concept for a trail, it is not my desire to take on the other two trails. I would most likely enjoy walking the Lake Champlain

Trail and would go crazy trying to enjoy a bike ride on the Hudson River Greenway trail. I would certainly try to bike the Hudson River Greenway trail were as my focus would not be to get in a fitness ride. Now I do understand from a commute standpoint the New York trail would make total sense for a user and their desire to travel from point A to point B, such as for work or to visit someone.

As you can see, these are very reasonable and understandable different three P ideals and presence of one, two, three provided with each different environment. The common item I am referencing is the effort to enjoy a good bike ride or cycling event for yourself while during the entire time you are making use of your smell, sight, and hearing to capture your ride perception, perspective, and perceived enjoyment.

Another area of importance I like to note regarding your development and understanding for the three Ps skill set development is an especially important and convenience vehicle used throughout the world. The use of this convenience item promoted a forever industry change and made several impacts on the world economy, environmental impact, and fuel technology.

The creation of cars, also known as automobiles, promoted a direct need to understand and develop your usage and need to become sharp minded with being proficient with your ability to grow and evolve with driving skills and actually become mature with operating an automobile. There is a hidden subconscious effort within yourself that either accepts the desire to be an active automobile user and/or will not be an automobile user.

Should you choose to learn to drive and become a licensed driver, your three P development and focus with understanding presences of one, two, three is critical. I say this because once you accept that you wish to become an automobile operator, you also must accept the responsibilities that are present with operating a vehicle. This acceptance is a direct relation with your ability to succeed and flourish as a driver and make use of your skill set daily. In fact it is to your best interest to become the best driver you can possibly be in order to survive the negative concerns that are associated with being an active driver. It is our goal to travel and return home safely every single day, and as a driver, there are mishaps you encounter all the time, and many of them is not because of your effort, instead it could be caused by other drivers' lack of usage of acknowledging the rule of perception, prospective, and perceived activities that he or she can avoid or control.

As a driver, we spend most of our time looking forward and the remaining of our time constantly processing the presence of one, two, three while in motion when driving. The presence of one, two, three when driving consists of acknowledging your **perception** of distance and timing, your **prospective** of what direction other vehicle are doing and watching directional signage and traffic lights alone with constantly processing data to keep your **perceived** calculations and assumptions active. When driving there is no order to how you process the three P understanding when operating an automobile. When you are at a stop, parked, or moving at various speeds, you are automatically shuffling the order of the three Ps and making major decisions along your route. When you are driving in the city, you adjust to what is present around you that consist of more tight and close contact, potential with pedestrians, vehicles, and structures such as the curbs or debris in the road or even potholes.

The automobile industry has created standards to aid in your ability to maintain your three P skill set, such as lighting and mirrors, including the actual automobile instrumentation systems. This all have direct interactions with your usage and practice of controlling and alone with having a positive and safe driving experience. As a society, the automobile industry have an obligation and regulation guidelines to promote positive experience with driving. They integrate technology to assist your three Ps usage. Unfortunately there still is a skill set that you must practice on your own with becoming a safe driver and operator of a vehicle.

Manual operation skill development is a must…When you are in motion, you are criticized if you fail to understand time and distance. You are also criticized if you avoid driving rules and do not practice good courtesy to others and respect the sharing of the roads. The most used tools when driving, in my opinion, to help you process the presence of one, two, three/three Ps is your skill set to make good use of looking in your side and review mirrors alone with controlling your speed.

The skill set development will allow you to make judgement with accident avoidance, give right of way to other drivers and allow you to change lanes, stop, or speed up so that you are not wrapped up in another driver's defaults or failure to promote good driving practices.

Over time you will become greatly confident with your ability to guide your influence on other drivers and maximize your safety efforts with driving.

A fire chief provides guidance and leadership at the scene of an emergency as he is responsible for directing the activities of the fire fighters and usage of equipment during real time. The fire chief makes use of his three Ps at every call for duty. He must process existing conditions while make use of his experience and real time assessment. While in route to the scene, the Fire Chief is preparing and processing his three Ps. He remembers they needed details from the initial call to duty and the nature of the call, which could be a car accident, a workplace incident, a rescue mission, or an actual fire.

In either of the cases, the fire chief is trained and make use of his experience and resources to provide leadership qualities at the onsite event. He also is responsible with making sure that he is aware of his team skill set and ready to make commands to achieve the best possible outcome while maintaining safety measures for all his reports and other involved parties during an emergency event.

Let's go through some common steps that the Chief will process with respect to how he is going to process the presence of one, two, three/three Ps as they will be shaped in a missed order.

Frist, he received a call to duty that provided him with data regarding the nature of the needed response. He also starts to format his perception as to what the scene may be based on the reports being provided to him by the dispatcher. Also based on his experience, he is starting to process his prospective before he arrives on the location.

Once he arrives, he is now ready to make commands based on his predetermined three Ps and now his actual on-site real-time assessment. The fire chief will blend his thoughts so that he can start addressing the emergency issued. He is also skilled to remain open minded to potential change in direction due to unforeseen conditions and new information provided to him by his team or the event will pronounce concerns that will need to be addressed.

- Physical Sight In the Field

- Smell & Sight of Food

- Fireman Prospective To A Fire Smell & Sight & Sounds

- Soldiers At / In War

- Driving

- TV & News

- Sounds What You Hear Guide Your 3P's IE Education & Learning

- A Person Physical Condition Football & Basketball, Other Sports

- Advertising via Smell

- Fitness

- Health & Doctor Reviews

- Anticipation Factor

- Disruption

- Truth In Systems

- Navigation Changes (Water Depth and Location)

Chapter 4

The True Reality and Balance

Vetting information to quality facts, important
Elements and values in order to include the right
Or proper understanding, expectations and needed
Awareness of the elements with the subject matter

Define Balance for the Chapter

The art of troubleshooting requires skill set that may consist of focus training session or experience in a particular field of interest or on how to handle a particular event that engages with one's skill set. With most troubleshooting efforts, it is necessary to prove the source of the fault or identify needed measure for resolve. Depending on the topic of discussion or subject of thought, there may be a need for testing or other proof of needed next step measure to identify the next step in a process to identify the root cause of the matter or topic at hand. In most of these cases, it is important to not conclude with were the issue or subject rest when considering the three Ps. Should there be a predetermine conclusion of the three Ps without taking the proper steps to assess the situation, the decided outcome may have short falls with the needed facts. In other words, it is particularly important to create a comprehensive investigation and review of the issue or subject matter in order to have proper progress regarding identification of the actual truth and fault before a solution can be implemented.

Let us use the world of science at this moment to highlight the importance of understanding this chapter subject of how to determine the true reality and balance. The focus is to make sure you take a solid understanding of process within your own approach when working to address the three Ps with respect to having your own comfort level with balance to identify the true reality when handling an issue, subject matter, or need to troubleshoot. Over the years, teams have shared best practices and means to review needed truth in the world of science on many fronts. There are established systematic methods based on proven evidence to determine facts, which are considered true reality in many situations and include secondary measures to support the truth, which are proven test and methods. Within the troubleshooting practice when proven two reasons why something is broken helps to assure the proper corrective actions. In short the definition of science is the use of scientific measures to determine the general truth. This short definition is clear to state a couple key point regarding true reality and offer an open-ended understanding on what is needed to establish a balance and comparable assessment. Because of this open-ended statement, there is need to have secondary measures to have an acceptable truth of reality when trying to determine the actual facts. It is human nature to hunt for the truth or facts and sometimes not accept the truth or fact while efforts at times to discount the facts. With science it is particularly important to conclude facts at a high level in order to have actual resolve.

Now let us touch on a different area regarding the need to have true reality in order to complete balance understanding and acceptance of the three Ps. This subject is well-studied and offers tones of data and is especially important to the world existence. This area of discussion or overview is weather forecasting.

The weather forecasting has a very direct impact on the three Ps in many areas of focus. As an individual, the weather impact your entire day with regards to how you travel, how you dress, and how you plan events regarding outdoor or indoor activities.

The weather forecast impact business, such as lawncare services, work to be completed on scaffold and lifting cranes. Scaffold and lifting crane work activities do not complete work on very windy or rainy days due to safety hazards standards. In addition, when it is very cold or extremely hot, certain activities are not completed, such as outdoor construction that involves concrete pouring. We avoid going to the beach when it is very cold or very windy and we like to go to the beach when it is warm and humid.

Our perception or attitude are heavily influenced by the weather forecast where we tend to feel upbeat and energized at our own desired climate conditions that is forecasted and plan our activities accordingly. For some people, they tend to feel dark and gloomy when the weather is not in their satisfaction range.

Your prospective and future outlook is dependent of the weather forecast; this can be a day to day prospective or a five-day look ahead where you agree or disagree how you will spend your time and activities based on the potential conditions of the weather.

The likelihood of your perceived conscious is formatted based on the weather forecast. This is a learned behavior that impacts your individual awareness with how you will govern yourself with the weather forecast.

Both the understanding of general science and weather forecasting provide us with two areas of how important it is to take time and understand what history has provided, how proven measures have determine the need to acknowledge the focus of needed acceptance of true reality and the balance of facts that governs the outcome. In most of everything we do, there is a positive and negative element hovering the subject matter or topic. For the purpose of understanding and minimize the negative impact, it is best of interest to develop your projection skill sets and take the time to use proven approaches to gather acceptance of reality and decide how you wish to move forward with your approach to balance.

Also, when processing the points of this chapter to enhance your conception and practice of true reality and balance, it is also to your advantage to develop your skill with monitoring practices to sustain your balance. You will need to address the cause for changes, need to modify and establish consistency with the facts of the reality you are dealing with in real-time or at some sort of interval. This practice will ensure your comfort levels and promote a positive outcome.

Monitoring and monitoring tools are a great way to keep track of changes and need to adjust. Your three Ps development in this area of identifying truth and fairness will provide you major self-enhancements with addressing real-time needed feedback or awareness with items that concern you or even when you need to implement this concept in your personal life or workplace. Monitoring can be a hard tools, such as electronics devices, or based on your skill set, you will establish your own tools within your judgement to promote a level of comfort through observations, thought, and qualification measures that are acceptable means to settle a decision or next stop efforts.

This is quite common with professional services, such as lawyers, doctors, engineers, or even a flight attendant. For example an experienced flight attendant has seen routine patterns over and over with respect to their observation of people boarding a plane, departing a plan, seating while in flight, and how they conduct themselves during a flight. The flight attendant through their observation gathers many three Ps about each person in every seat once they are seated. They can assess and determine if a passenger or passengers are traveling as an individual with a group or even have some sort of association with the travel of the flight for a person that can be related to a vacation or business trip. Also, while in flight, the flight attendant makes decisions regarding how to comfort you while in flight. If you have children in fight, they are prepared to cater to the needs of a child based on continue observation, judgement, and experience. If the passage is an older person who have movement concerns, they are there to interact with others on your behalf to assure your comfort while in flight.

Using my viewpoint here, the flight attendant prospective I am sharing provides an interesting viewpoint to touch base on with respect to secondary care of others projection or experiences with the three Ps. The flight attendant as a professional is proving each passenger, which are millions of people, over a course of a year with advance support of your inflight positive exposure of your travel expectations. They are there to do their best to assure that you have a positive outlook (prospective), meet your anticipations (perceived), and maintain a good attitude (perception) during your flight and interaction with the entire travel. They are there to help avoid misperceptions, wrong impressions, and dismal experiences for the entire inventory of people during the flight. This is a large undertaken that requires acceptance for control balance of needs for everyone and assurance of your travel reality. How often do you hear the question, "How was your flight?" from someone once you have safely arrived at your destination?

This is a quite common question that target your response to express and share your feedback in reference to your flight experience. Was your flight experience acceptable to your three Ps is the core inquire being suggested. Was the reality of your trip a good balanced feeling for you as an individual or group, and also the underline question here has a hidden core point that is important which is was there any concerns that needed to be address or was it addressed by the flight attendant.

There are also some common somewhat negative responses regarding flight experiences, such as "The landing was a little bumpy, my flight was one hour late" or "the captain did not provide good flight updates."

When discussing the subject of balance, it is my personal practice to review both sides of a subject or issue when practices the three Ps. So some of the positive responses to share when ask the question regarding your flight can be "I had a smooth on-time flight, the in-flight service was great" and "The captain provided perfect weather and arrival time feedback."

These are important information that enlighten your off-boarding mood once you are on the ground and transitioning from the airplane. Your mood is important and have a direct foundation of your three Ps grasp and appreciation. Your interpretation of your flight summary is your reality and that cannot be changed. In fact you feel compelled to complete a survey form to share your experience so that management can review your experience to suggest needed improvement or advise comments that help with service housekeeping.

Quality control have a true reality and balance interface where the process is created to gain review factors and elements that defines integrity. In business, customer service, or in your personal life, you want to understand how you shape your quality control and delivery when interacting with others or in your lifestyle. Yes…There is a difference between your lifestyle and environments outside of your personal life. In general, in order to have a healthy formation of your own mindset with shaping your thoughts and values, it is to your interest to shape your internal system that welcomes tools that enhances your complete fulfillment and self-standards.

Regardless of what professional services that are being performed, there is a strong desire to maximize the desire outcome and hold nothing back so that you received a high level of satisfaction and comfort. This also applies to how you like to output others acceptance of your efforts when you are in the lead role to perform or provide a high level of entrusted experience to an induvial or group. These are core facts that I am suggesting to be a part of your three Ps development. It is classy and magnificent once you can automate yourself to have a subconscious timely recognition with identifying and shaping your influence of quality control awareness.

The material that you generate defines your ability to captivate support of the truth alone with establishing genuineness have great value. You will in most cases win over individuals and groups because you have provided them with strong belief and sense of positive three Ps. This is how business and individuals can have long-term relationships with others over a long period of time. The three Ps are in a positive position with all involved and the process of maintaining balance, reality alone with quality control measures establishes consistence interactions and trust.

Surveillance efforts is a solid subject that promotes balance to gain real existents opposed to subjective guessing as to what the truth may be regarding what is being monitored. This tool of surveillance offers detail qualification of the needed or unknown information that is being gathered. It is critical that the needed material is obtained in order to comment your understanding as to how you settle your thought or next step and act on your own perspective, perception, and acceptance of our perceived belief.

The video surveillance market and industry is projected to be worth $86.5 billion by 2027 according to market analysis. The core drivers for this growth is due to video surveillance systems usage in commercial infrastructure, public places, private and residential buildings.

The three Ps is again in full concept when working to assure unbiased feedback and raised the level of assurance regarding the true reality and balance subject of this chapter. Marketing is amazingly simple with this technology as there is a strong demand for monitoring and the video surveillance market is proving to support how on a global level that this tool make help vetting needed information to identify actual positive or negative feedback to the three Ps. In fact, on many platforms, it is mandatory to install surveillance equipment to remove doubt and encourage monitoring in order to have proactive measure for the three Ps.

The information provided through surveillance measures is critical and have lasting monetary or legal positioning factors to protect an asset, provide proactive security and real-time monitoring.

When you watch the local news and television and a crime has taken place in modern times, one of the first and automatic evidence shown is a video surveillance clip that promotes a pronounce three P implant in the minds of viewers. They are more powerful than a picture or photo because the video data provide data if the data was not altered. Steps and other technology tools are in place to vet video surveillance data should the information is needed for law enforcement or other needs for vetting video data. Regardless for the purpose of true reality and balance, this technology is a great example. Other similar tools are voice recorders, motion detectors, and vibration devices, which are used in areas where the end users wish to be informed to pronounce three Ps (prospective, perceived, and perception) findings should an item being monitor have been breached and require physical inspection, such as an area that have glass protection of jewelry or a large production motor that is working outside of its design vibration tolerance. Vibration technology are common monitoring or surveillance tools for expensive machinery, including aircraft machines and space rockets.

Without doubt or with respect to a high level of understanding, reality is a form of perception belief that either was proving or belief in theory that such a matter is true. Based on your perception of the reality, truth or not, your subconscious forms your prospective and perceived ideals. Assumption is minimized when you can complete detail observation of activities to help manage the truth and the related goals. The information helps shape the three Ps so that a next step of action can be supported and completed. The intent is to require a positive desired outcome.

The FBI commonly use profiling measures to help with their cases to resolve crime. This is also a form of true reality and balance determination process that is a proving crime science practice by the Federal Bureau of Investigation under the term crime science, which studies crime events to gather facts related to three Ps net results. These results are confirmed environmental crime facts, behavior, and patterns.

They can spend a lot of man hours and resources gathering information to establish or improve upon a case three Ps. Very often the effort will change several times before the team advance their efforts.

Crime profiling in the area of law enforcement that fall under two areas I like to mention, which are criminal profiling that focus on the personality and characteristics of an offender. The second topic is crime scene profiling, which focus on the elements described at the physical scene that capture the scene tendencies, demographic variables to format a possible model for reference. This may also offer some emotional observations of the offender. However, both profiling practices by law enforcement, including the FBI, have a degree of bias and distort components that require vetting to establish reality. Just like all things that have open ended information or unresolved data, the subject remains open for interpretation, causing imbalance with the needed three P resolve establish within the law enforcement platform.

It is extremely important to get matters resolved and assure that an offender have broken a rule of law and evidence that will support charges towards a crime is permissible in order to process the three Ps and gain legal support. There are many cases involving sex or serial murder crimes that have taken lengthy timelines to satisfy criminal trail hearings that lead to convictions. These trail hearings are the presentation of findings, which are results of negative prospective, perceived, and perception feedback arguments that being vetting in order to hold the offender accountable for their actions.

There is a general argument that is ongoing where anti-realism is formed because reality or the lack of balance is being promoted to accept particle proven reality situations or subject matter. In other words, anti-realism is a denial of the truth or one taking a position not to believe in the topic or essence that is in discussion or being work on that can be between individuals or a group.

One should take a long time to themselves to understand how you will self-govern yourself with how you identify the truth, how you monitor and balance the position you wish to take on a given matter while being diplomatic, or winning over others to reach goals and advance.

We all want to make popular decision versus unpopular decision; this goes hands and hand with gaining support or losing support, including positive and negative three Ps. *Reminder as you read through the three P concept, the goals is to provide readers with information so that you develop your own self-management and practice of the three Ps, meaning how you govern yourself and process perceived, prospective, and perception.* For this reason, taken time to assure facts is a major step to assure you are making the best decisions to next step your effort and assure a positive outcome.

It is ok to take time versus having pre-mature finalization that could cause major controllable backslash. Very often decisions are prolonged due to needed truth finding methods are introduce during the process. One of the common areas you see this is with a court trails where a lawyer may say to a Judge, "Your Honor, I have new evidence in this case, may I approach the bench?" The judge will in most cases accept the new findings and add more time to a trial in order to be open minded for the need to balance and have an open door for reality.

As regards to building a project that you wish to be successful, there are truth finding and reality measure completed to determine check and balance systems to assure you are making corrections or adjusting to what is needed to assure the desire outcome or building for additional success. Again vetting practices and procedures come in different forms, and as we continue to review the three Ps and your effort to establish your own mindset and ways you install tools to develop your knowledge or skill, set it to your best of interest to learn additional tools that enable you to identify details to enlighten your success effort. These can be learned behaviors on your behalf alone with reusable tools. The ideal to reinforced, your ability to show or share the true reality with balance to win over others or progress your effort requires not just talk but supporting materials to advance your goals.

Depending on the nature of the project, work, or discussion you are involved in, which can be presented as a model that provide a representation of an object or system in order to review or capture important facts or expectations. In the clothing or garment industry, physical people models are used to demonstrate fashion designs were three Ps are expression by the physical women or men models that complete a series of runway walk through were by standers can actual have a straightforward prospective of the clothing wear or outfit in addition to having the opportunity to touch and feel the product. The audience can also gain a perception with how the garment may fit on different body styles and able to perceive if they choose to make a purchase of the product that may lead to project potential sales.

Prototype is an advance model or modeling process where you can incorporate more components into a model or product that have more moving parts and components. Machinery is an example as to why an actual prototype will provide precision details as to how, what, and why a particular design will provide the reality or performance that the mission or concept is trying to achieve. The prototype approach and platforms are a serious research and development tool for many manufacturing companies to qualify their work and design intent. Within your effort to create a balance with findings and acceptance with the truth, think about how you can insert this as prototype understanding into your situation or extend the time, including fact finding efforts.

Structural engineers complete a lot of projects using concrete as a source to build and support buildings, bridges, roads, and load barring support members, such as concrete columns. For their fact-finding effort, they use a process to determine the strength of existing concrete to determine the facts about the concrete strength, moisture content/level, including other orientation factors that are needed in civil engineering design task in order to assure that the concrete can perform and support weight and a fixture lifecycle. The process is a global practice and support by American Society for Testing and Materials (ASTM). ASTM is an international standards organization that publishes technical standards for products, materials, and systems so that credibility truths are maintain throughout the world. This is a necessary reality needed so that items, such as concrete performance, can support its design intent. Once a structure is built or during the building process, three Ps' efforts must be qualitied in order to assure no issues with structure defects, including a short life space for what was built or supported by concrete.

In simple terms, at the end of each day, we want the true reality and balance to have a firm concrete form in order to remove bias issues and provide support for the reality that we desire. This is a good metaphor to how serious it is and important to establish your self-management and use of tools to assure you have a high level of usage to assess, evaluate, or appraise your study to identify truth and reality of any item you are concern with or exercise leadership liaison role within a work group to earn your respect or enhance your representation role within a team.

- Hate Books

- Perception was ignored or silence.

- Marketing & Research

- Where there is smoke, there is fire

- Perception is Reality comment Bias Promotion.

- Projection

- Weather Forecasting

- Monitoring or Bench Marking

- List Vehicles (Models, Prototype, Core Samples Test

- Maintain Status or Self Status

- Construction Design

- Understanding Threats

- Planting (good seed and soil versus influence of anger, resentfulness, selfishness) & Harvesting & Atmosphere Environment (sin neg and positive) , Storm vs Reality

- Pure Truth Can Control The Storm You Can Control Your Steering

- Follow Advise Manage3 Voyage

Chapter 5

Breaking Down The Argument

Take time to set up and review the facts, elements
Or influences of the subject matter. Allow others to
Express their 3-Ps than follow up with backcheck and
Set agreement. If needed circle back after completing

Research and additional information.

Similar to my earlier flooding event at a high-end hotel in Washington DC were the general manager had his own understanding or lack of understanding on how to address needed water supply for his hotel during a mayor's convention, I have found myself in debates or arguments regarding facility design changes, and it is required of me to explain the core and roots of issues, including needed resolve and how the situation or event arrived at this undesired state. It is quite common that design concepts are created and fall short of needed details to achieve the overall long-term function or desired impact. In addition, during the design stages, a team of people such as engineers, design architect, and the customer have concept discussions. During these discussions, normally a team is sent to survey the site conditions or area of concern to develop renderings models or test fit plans to use as a base to create a broader idea for what the overall design will turn out to be and then add finishes and resources to support those finishes.

This particular project concept I was involved with was to be complete, a lobby redesign and change the exterior row of canopies. The canopies were overhead covering at several doors for the entrance of the building outlet, which consist of a couple food outlets, office building main entrance, and an office supply retail store.

The canopy design involved the change from an old dated non-attractive metal arrangement to an updated anodized aluminum finishes that matches other local building cosmetic exterior appearance with a rich shining metal. The look actually provided the site with a improve elegance appearance and was inviting for general public. The main entrance had a revolving door with two side entrance doors that is a part of the scope of work to be change to new glass panel herculite doors.

Once the project was completed, there were major issues with the lobby temperature control that cause the lobby to be very cold when the outside temperatures were below the freezing point. Alone with wind gust, the lobby could not reach an acceptable temperature. It is particularly important to have a lobby of a building at acceptable temperatures, which is one of the first impressions of a facility main lobby. The main lobby is an area where its occupants and guests gather and set a tone for welcoming, greeting, or an important meeting. It is also a location for when you enter a facility you have removed yourself from the outdoor elements.

I was called into a meeting to discuss the issue regarding the excessive cold lobby temperatures. The management team started to focus on the lack of preventative maintenance for the two heat and air conditioning units that supported the lobby climate control. The on-site team of engineers completed on time routine preventative maintenance to the units per the preventative maintenance schedule. I advise the team at the table that the design changes for the lobby promoted a major defect with the design and scope of work. Because the management team created what they thought is a positive cosmetic enhancement change to the main lobby, it was a creative change and refreshing look for the site, however they did not detail the engineering concerns. It is also quite common that engineering items or review of the scope of work is omitted. The concept of deferring engineering items from a scope of work is call Removal of Valued Engineering (VE). Value engineering is an organized methodical approach with providing the steps or functions to a project to reduce cost.

The practice to promote value engineering to a project on the surface save money and reduce project cost on the front end and become falsely attractive to the those who focus on saving money. Once a project is complete, in many cases a post project argument is created. These arguments are mostly fact-finding inspections or evaluations to identify root cause for the defective design issue. It is also incredibly sad that the original design concepts become the ownership of the induvial that sign off on the project and refuse to accept the project short falls.

One of the tactics when having an open argument, the drivers of the argument tend to insert diversions, false perceptions that also provide unsupported perceive information to gain support. The drivers who are building these false perceptions and unsupported data, which is perceives information gain believe and momentum for their object to avoid ownership. Once they establish these base lines, they tend to build on that perception to others. Now the argument is established, and within human nature alone with fast tracking of time, a group or individual wants to close the finalize a project. In this instance, the misbelieved focus was lack of preventative maintenance as to why the lobby was very cold during the low temperature winter months.

All involved who believe these negative three Ps are now ready to focus on how they need to improve the preventative maintenance program versus listen to what facts were discovered and found to be the core issues with the project design, which was a VE (Valued Engineering) practice to save funds that resulted in a long-term issue. Valued engineering practices are attractive regarding short-term understanding and provide a long-term issue.

As I provide my life experience on why I am encouraged to share the three Ps concept and develop your own style with processing issues and topics, this chapter "Breaking Down The Argument". No one wants to be at fault for a short fall with a project, and those who are sincere will admit to the issue and avoid casting blame on others. They will break down the issue or argument by vetting the true information. The long-term desire in most cases for a project of this nature was to provide a positive experience for its guest and occupants. The design team not only had an issue during the winter months. There was also a core issue during the summer months where the lobby would be the total opposite of being very cold to being very hot in the summer. A hot lobby in the summer is just as bad as a cold lobby in the winter. Here is a three Ps overview…Imagine taking a six-block walk in the cold from the nearest subway station at eight degrees outside under a high wind gust, which promotes a wind chill factor on your body. Then arriving to a cold lobby and getting no relief before you either go to your workstation or a meeting. Your perception was once you arrive at the building, you would warm up, get comfortable in a few minutes, be ready to conduct business. This was also your prospective once you started walking in the cold eight degrees that you would weather the elements until you get to the lobby of the building and then get relief and comfort once you are inside. In the summertime, after walking eight blocks from a subway station when the temperature is ninety degrees and the relative humidity is over sixty, your perception is once you reach the lobby, you can stop sweating, sit in the lobby, and gather yourself to prepare to take care of business or go to your work station. Instead you are sweating and uncomfortable and need to go to the rest room to wash down with a paper towel before your meeting.

The lobby climate control issue will continue during periods of extreme humid hot days and extremely low cold temperatures and especially noted in both cases of hot or low temperatures that also have an active wind gust. The wind gust forces the exterior climate condition elements into the lobby space faster, which further hinder the original air conditioning and heating system design capacity to either catch up or run extra-long time in order to attempt to reach a comfortable temperature for the lobby space.

The gaps in the new herculite doors remain the root issue. There was substantial disagreement from the owner representatives with the fact that the existing air conditioning and heating system could not keep up after proving unit performance was at its maximum capacity. The designers were open minded to adding supplement heating to the entrance doorway, which would precondition the air at the entrance before entering the lobby space. They would add a heater in the vestibule space. This is the space between the outside entrance and before the second set of interior herculite doors.

Because of project pride or being fixated on the initial design concept, the decision makers who supported the original design did not want to acknowledge the change to make right and improvement to the needed HVAC climate control needed to assure what was best for the long-term. This concern needed revisit of the scope of work and would involve a change order and needed funding. Also, with this change order, a discussion to upper management regarding the project cost overage would need to be explained and justified. This is a discussion that was being avoided.

During another project that had a major short fall with its scope of work, the project was local government enforced issue for a hotel ability to cook and provide food to its customers. The kitchen of a major hotel had a grease fire in the kitchen due to poor kitchen hood exhaust. The system was dated and had poor maintenance. The local fire department responded to the site to put out the fire. It is common practice for city fire department to follow up with post fire investigation to determine origin and cause. The city fire department completed their report and ordered the hotel to upgrade the kitchen hood system. The hotel completed cleaning of the exhaust hood system and performed repairs to assure that the existing system was operational to satisfy the Fire Marshall for the short-term, which allow the hotel to continue to make use of the current system and keep services open until the upgrade was completed.

Now that the hotel was on record to upgrade the kitchen hood system by the local fire department Fire Marshall office, the management team was forced to commit to making this needed improvement. This type of project for a business operation requires professional services, such as an outside consultant firm to provide detail plans and scope of work. These plans and scope of work are then packaged in a request for bid document and forward to general contractors to provide cost estimates for the project. General contractors have a common practice to provide estimate based on the information provided if they are not doing the design work themselves. During the request for prices or bidding process, all general contractors typically price or bid the same, provided bidding information to them and the other bidders. They will ask questions for clarification known as Request For Information (ROI) and share this information with all other bidders so that all the bidders are seeing, sharing, and providing prices for the same scope of work. If they are not providing price for the same scope of work, the entire effort would be incomplete and need to start all over, making sure that all bidders have the same information. The common simple terms use to express like for like bidding is called comparing apples to apples.

The intent is to make sure that reasonable documentation and understanding of the scope of work as a clear and providing like for like comparison, so that the prices for the scope of work match up for an award decision to the contractor of choice that show that they captured the scope of work and able to complete the work at the cost provided. Just like in the lobby door changes the owner or design team did not want to see large change orders after a project that have been priced, bid, and awarded.

In most cases…Yes…A change order needs to be supported and funded in order to complete the project on time and is best for the long-term. The argument is that magic question of "Why did we not see that before."

Project management is an art, a profession that require effort and experience alone with making sure the right players or consultant groups are involved with the desire concept, design, or issue that is being addressed. With the kitchen hood upgrade project, the Fire Marshall notice advises an upgrade to the kitchen hood system. The hotel management team took this notice and contacted a Mechanical Engineer Group to review the system and recommend needed upgrade. The Mechanical Engineering Group completed a survey and recommended a kitchen hood replacement to the hotel management.

The hotel management took this recommendation and presented this as a resolved to the upper management team for approval. The estimated noted in the mechanical engineering group recommendation was $15,000 for a new kitchen hood. This recommendation satisfied what the hotel management team thought was the needed resolve, and they just need to bid the project out to mechanical contractors and complete the needed upgrade. The funds were approved for $15,000 and noted in the hotel capital project improvement plan.

Once I was on board with the management team, I inherited the kitchen hood project alone with another capital improvement project to replace the cooling tower that was on a lower floor surrounded by hotel guest rooms. The cooling tower was causing guests to complain about the noise of the mechanical equipment especially at night. This cooling tower issue was captured on the guest satisfaction survey as an ongoing complaint. The survey is a good practice and offer great three P feedback.

Those who study guest satisfaction feedback using the different formats and platforms is an outstanding illustration of the importance gathering data (perceived feedback), guest experiences (combination of prospective and perception).

Now that I am on the job and received the capital improvement file, which contain the project's cost and scope of work I in turn reviewed this information and start to format the plan to execute contracts language and schedules to complete the upgrade. I notice that the kitchen hood project have very large short falls with the scope of work needed to complete the project successfully and noted concerns not to disturb the normal operations of the hotel. The kitchen hood that was sited by the fire department was in the main kitchen area where all the food for the restaurants, banquet service and other major food preparations for the hotel is conducted. It is important to exhaust fumes from cooking activities so that the indoor air quality of the hotel is comfortable for people on the inside of the building. Poor air quality can cause discomfort, such as nausea, vomiting, and respiratory breathing concerns.

As I continue my project management planning, it is also my practice to walk the space and path of the project from a physical perspective so that I can gather my understanding of the three Ps (project prospective, perceived workflow, and activity perception). This is important so that needed communication, adjustments, and impact on others can be captured in advance.

As I move about with my walk through with the reading of the scope of work in mind, I started taking notes of issues that impacted the full needed scope of work. Also, as an engineer, it is my responsibility and job knowledge to understand building codes, local ordinance, and risk management concerns with planning a project. The hotel had dated building materials, fire alarm system, and needed a temporary kitchen so that the impact on the overall food services operation would not be interrupted and needed to be addressed. Can you image a hotel telling its guests that we will not be able to provide food services for the in room food orders, breakfast, lunch, dinner, and banquets events due to the kitchen hood project that will take weeks to complete? NO… This would be unacceptable and impact the hotel ability to make revenue and income due to the project, let alone promote short falls with the forecast of income due to guest are set to arrive through the reservations system during the project construction period. As a project manager in a hotel operation, you never want to disturb the reservation forecast. This will cause huge heartburns with the subject of "Breaking Down the Argument". The ideal is to control what you can thorough planning, so that there is no argument to break down. For example, with hotels, since we are on the subject, when there are projects to upgrade the guest rooms, we project managers or planners discuss this with the reservation team and remove rooms from inventory and place rooms back in inventory to meet reservations expectations. This also applies for the use of the banquet and meeting rooms space. The finance team in turn are not able to not forecast revenue income and the sales team are aware that they cannot book sales during the construction or project timeframe.

Now that I have identified the short falls with the needed scope of work, I can now add information needed to develop the scope of work and associated cost. Once this is completed and double checked for accuracy, I can now explain the project details to upper management. As a manager, it is my practice to update information weekly and share my progress regarding justification of project status and related information for projects that are in progress.

The Kitchen Hood project original budget was $15,000, and after my review and project update, the project actual cost was over $900,000. I am sure that this create a major argument of my findings and my preparations to explain the cost which amount to an overage of 98 percenr from the original project cost.

The fact that I now must tell the hotel local management team that their original project was only 2 percent the scope of work and to hear me explain that the project needed an additional 98 percent scope of work increase was very disturbing. I recall having a meeting with a senior manager that flew in town to meet with me to discuss my findings. He advised me that I was way over budget. I remain calm and settle during our discussion. I advise him that the project was understated and that the 98 percent was their choice to make or just move forward with 2 percent effort of $15,000 and not satisfy the Fire Marshall office.